Before It Was Too Late

Before It Was Too Late

A true story of pancreatic disease, cardiac crisis,

and the power of acting early

Peter R. Mittler

I did not know how close I was to dying

until I was already on the path to survival

This book is a work of personal experience and reflection. It is not intended to provide medical advice, diagnosis, or treatment. Readers should seek the advice of qualified medical professionals regarding their own health conditions.

Every effort has been made to ensure the accuracy of the information contained in this book. However, medical knowledge and recommendations change over time, and the author makes no representations or warranties regarding completeness or applicability to individual circumstances.

First edition
Perth, Western Australia

ISBN: 978-1-7645686-2-3
Paperback edition
Printed by Amazon KDP

Cover design and interior layout by Peter Robert Mittler

10 9 8 7 6 5 4 3 2 1

This book is dedicated to all those who lost their lives to
pancreatic cancer
some without ever knowing it was there.

People whose symptoms were subtle,
whose warning signs were quiet,
and whose time to act passed unseen.

May greater awareness help others
recognise the signs earlier,
ask harder questions,
and seek answers while there is still time.

In memory of some well-known lives lost to
pancreatic cancer:

Steve Jobs
Alex Trebek
Patrick Swayze
Alan Rickman
Ruth Bader Ginsburg
Luciano Pavarotti
John Hurt
Sally Ride
Tony Esposito (Chicago Blackhawks)
my MG Car Club of Toronto friend, Jon Rosenthall

...and the countless others whose names are known
only to their families and friends.

Awareness saves time.

Time saves lives—before it is too late.

Introduction

Read This First

If you don't read the entire book, that's understandable. Life is busy.

But please read these three pages.

This book is about how I almost died—and why I didn't.

This is a story about timing, awareness, and the consequences of waiting too long.

Health stories can feel heavy. Sometimes we simply don't have the time or energy to take in someone else's journey.

But these three pages might save your life.

What follows is not medical advice. It is simply what happened to me. Looking back, there were warning signs, decisions, delays, and moments where acting sooner rather than later made all the difference.

A Timeline of What Happened:

2018 — First Episode
While visiting in Perth, Australia, I experienced acute pancreatitis. It was painful and frightening, but at the time it seemed like an isolated event.

2018–2020 — Recurring Episodes
The pancreatitis returned. Tests were done. Imaging

became more concerning. Specialists began to talk about long-term risks.

Spring 2020 — A Critical Decision
I was advised to consider a total pancreatectomy to prevent cancer before it had a chance to develop. It was not an easy decision, but waiting carried its own risks.

July 2020 — Major Surgery During COVID-19
My pancreas was removed. Recovery was difficult and complicated, and I began learning how to live as a brittle diabetic.

July 2020 — An Unexpected Threat
During recovery, doctors discovered that my heart was in serious danger. I had severe coronary blockage that had produced few clear symptoms.

July 2020 — A Heart Attack and Another Decision
I suffered a cardiac event and faced another major decision—whether to proceed with high-risk bypass surgery.

Autumn 2020 — Recovery and a Second Chance
Against long odds, I survived. Recovery was slow, humbling, and life-changing.

I am here to tell the story.

And the story might help save your life too.

Why I Am Telling This Story?

I was fortunate in many ways:

- I had access to skilled doctors.
- I had people who pushed me when I needed push ing.
- I had moments of clarity that helped me choose action instead of delay.

Not everyone gets those chances.

If something in your body feels wrong, persistent, or unexplained—

Don't wait.

Ask questions.

Seek another opinion if necessary.

Follow through on tests.

Act sooner rather than later.

The purpose of this book is not to frighten you.

It is to make you aware.

Because sometimes the difference between life and death is not medicine alone—it is timing.

Peter R. Mittler
Perth, Western Australia

Preface

This book began as a way to make sense of a sequence of events that unfolded over several years, across two countries, and through a period of modern history when hospitals became quieter, lonelier places.

In March 2018, I was in Perth, Australia, when I experienced acute pancreatitis—an episode that seemed, at the time, like a painful interruption that would resolve and be forgotten. It didn't. Over the next two years, the episodes returned, the imaging became more concerning, and the decisions in front of me narrowed. Eventually, a specialist said the words no one wants to hear: "total pancreatectomy." Remove the entire pancreas—before cancer arrived, before the window closed, before waiting became the most dangerous choice.

The surgery was scheduled for July 2020, during COVID-19. Like many people in that time, my family and I faced a version of medical crisis that carried an extra layer of isolation. Visitors were restricted. Ordinary support systems were unavailable. Much of what mattered happened through phone calls, FaceTime, and the steady presence of nurses and clinicians who did their work under pressure, behind masks, and within protocols that often felt both necessary and absurd.

I survived the surgery. Then I had a major heart attack.

The story that follows becomes, in some ways, less about illness and more about timing—about how quickly a situation can change, how fragile the margin can be, and how much depends on the people who notice small things early and act while action is still possible.

I have written this for a few reasons.

I wrote it:

- to honour the clinicians and doctors and nurses whose competence and humanity carried me through.
- for my family—Patty, our children, and the people who stood by us when they could not always be physically present. and
- for anyone who finds themselves living inside uncertainty, waiting for a call, waiting for a test result, waiting for a decision that cannot be comfortably delayed.

This is not a medical textbook, and I'm not a physician. It is a patient's account of what it felt like—emotionally, practically, and spiritually—to move through a long medical gauntlet and come out the other side changed. Where I describe medical events, I've tried to be as accurate as possible. If you are a medical student and want to read the clinical notes, contact me at pmittler@gmail.com and we can discuss it, and I can share it with you.

What I learned—slowly, repeatedly—is that survival is not only about the dramatic moments. It is often about the quiet ones: the decisions made early, the warning signs noticed, the small interventions taken in time. It is about the discipline of paying attention, and the courage to act before certainty arrives.

In the end, this is a story about care, timing, and blessed second chances.

And it all happened before it was too late.

—Peter Mittler

Acknowledgements

Patricia

There are some debts in life that cannot be repaid, only acknowledged with gratitude. Loving you is one of them.

You are my best friend, my soul mate, and my companion through every uncertain hour. Before the surgeries, during the long days in hospital, and through the slow and often difficult recovery, you were there—steady, calm, and quietly strong.

At the time, I did not fully grasp how close we came to losing the life we had built together. I was focused on surviving one day at a time. You carried the wider burden—the fear, the waiting, the unknown. The weight of that must have been immense, though you rarely let it show.

Your strength was not loud or dramatic. It was the strength of presence, of patience, of unwavering care. It was the strength that held everything together when I could not.

Years before all of this, I wrote a song for us called *"Thanks for Walking Down This Road With Me."* I did not realise then how true those words would become.

We walked that road together. And we are still walking it.

Julia

Our eldest daughter—the one who first made us parents.

It must have been very difficult to watch from Perth as we went through the trauma of surgeries, the near-death experience, and the long uncertainty of COVID-19. Distance can make worry even harder, because there is so little you can do except wait and hope.

We know you were as supportive as you could be from afar, and your love and encouragement meant a great deal to us during that time. A parent never forgets the quiet strength of a child who stands beside them, even at a distance.

Matthew

How helpless you must have felt. And how grateful I was that you dropped everything in Calgary to fly to Toronto to support your mother and me, only to be denied access to see me because of the COVID-19 shutdown.

Thank you for the two weeks you spent in Oshawa, waiting and supporting Mom while I remained in isolation. Your being there mattered more than you may ever know.

I am also deeply grateful to Jennifer, who capably and lovingly cared for your three boys as a single parent for those weeks, making it possible for you to be there when we needed you most.

Alyssa

When you were first born, Poppa Roy looked at you and said to me, *"This is the one who will care for you in your older days."*

At the time, I smiled and dismissed it as grandfatherly sentiment. I had no way of knowing how true those words would become.

Your years of nursing training at Trent University, followed by cardiac work in Sudbury as a perfusionist assistant and later paediatrics at SickKids, prepared you for a role neither of us could have foreseen.

Even across the distance—Perth to Toronto—you were there. You translated the language of medicine when it overwhelmed me and helped me understand what the doctors were saying, what the risks were, and what recovery would look like. That guidance meant more than you may ever know.

And you are still doing it today. Now that we are both in Perth, you keep a quiet, watchful eye on me—checking in, asking thoughtful questions, and noticing things I might otherwise overlook.

Thank you, not only for your professional knowledge, but for the care and love you have always given as my daughter.

To all our children and grandchildren, whose love, encouragement, and patience sustained us through those difficult months—thank you. Family is the thread that holds life together when everything else feels uncertain.

And so, with gratitude,
we keep walking the road ahead.

Table of Contents

Chapter 1: Nothing Odd, Right?

March 22–24, 2018

It started the way a lot of trouble starts — quietly, and after a particularly good week. We were in Perth, Australia, and we had been eating well. Fish and chips by the ocean. Pizza and beer. Red wine and steak. All the things your mother tells you not to eat, even though you know she'd have eaten them too.

Antacid tablets

Late one night — about 11:30 — I was chewing on the Australian equivalent of TUMS, something called 'Quick-Eze', trying to settle what I assumed was reflux. Normally two tablets would knock it out. This time, they didn't. That was unusual. Not alarming. Just… odd.

I said to Patricia, "I've got a pain just under my sternum."

She asked, "Is it in your chest?"

"No," I said. "More under my left rib cage."

"How's your heart rhythm?"

"Normal. Remember I fell off my bike a couple of weeks ago and landed hard on my ribs? They've been sore since then. But nothing like this."

She paused for about half a second and said, "We're going to the emergency department."

By the time we arrived at Joondalup Health Campus around 1:30 in the morning, my whole abdomen hurt. Not sharp pain — more like everything was wrong at once. I felt rotten.

I was admitted to the surgical unit and initially told it looked like a gallbladder attack. I was put on IV fluids and pain medication and told not to eat or drink anything — NPO, nothing by mouth — to give my system a chance to settle. [**NPO** comes from the Latin phrase *nil per os,* which literally means **"nothing through the mouth."**]

While I was lying there, waiting, my mind wandered to something completely unrelated: the travel insurance policy we buy every year before coming to Australia. Expensive? Yes. Necessary? Absolutely. The hospital required a thousand-dollar deposit on my American Express card.

To be honest, I didn't care.

Later that day, the surgeon came in. In Australia, surgeons are addressed as "Mr." rather than "Doctor," which somehow makes everything sound more serious.

Mr. Dorfman explained that my gallbladder ultrasound was perfectly clear. No stones. No sludge. Nothing.

"So, what is it?" I asked.

"You have acute pancreatitis," he said. "Your pancreatic duct is dilated — seven to ten millimetres — and twisted. It should be about three millimetres and smooth. I recommend you follow this up when you return to Canada."

I did not understand everything he said, but I did understand one thing: my close friend Jon Rosenthall had recently been diagnosed with late-stage pancreatic cancer. He had told me, more than once, that he wished someone had ordered an ultrasound a year earlier.

That stayed with me.

Chapter 2: Can You Fix It Fast?

May 2018

Back home in Canada, I booked a physical with my family doctor, Larry Bacher.

"Larry," I said, "I had a pancreatic attack in Perth, and I need you to take a serious look."

He was honest. "I'm not an expert on pancreatic disease, but let's get an MRI and see what's going on."

The MRI was scheduled for October. It was August.

That timing mattered more than anyone realised at first. We had a family cruise booked on the *Majestic Princess,* sailing from Auckland in December. To get there, we had to fly. Travel insurance could only be bought if there were no unresolved medical issues in the ninety days before travel. Any undiagnosed condition inside that window made insurance impossible.

There was fifty thousand dollars' worth of travel at stake — but more than that, there was the fact that this cruise was a rare gathering of our whole family. The idea that everyone would go without us was deeply unsettling

So, the clock was ticking.

I had imaging done at Lakeridge Health Centre in Oshawa on September 10, 2018. Waiting for the radiology report felt endless. When it finally came back, Larry referred me to his colleague, Dr. Tim Devlin, a gastroenterologist.

Looking back, I didn't understand then what I know now. The MRI showed a pancreatic duct that looked like a twisted telephone cord. Dilated. Irregular. That meant obstruction. And obstruction raises questions you don't want to ask too soon — especially the word cancer. The MRI images made the problem unmistakably clear.

Around the same time, I was watching Jon Rosenthall

deteriorate. His diagnosis had come late, and the disease was unforgiving. I arranged a special recognition award for him through the North American MGB Register, supported by John Twist. I also wrote and recorded a song called *He's a Certified MGB Nut* in his honour.

I told myself it was for Jon.

In truth, it was also for me.

Chapter 3: Hip, Hip, Hooray

September 2018

As if one medical situation weren't enough, Patty was dealing with her own. Throughout the summer of 2018, her left hip had been steadily getting worse. After multiple visits to the Holland Orthopaedic Clinic at Sunnybrook, it became clear that surgery before our December travel date was unlikely.

On September 4th, we called Maria — Dr Ravi's co-ordinator — to ask if there was any chance of a surgery date before our flight.

"Not a chance," she said.

The final cruise payment was due September 18th. Once that was paid, we were committed.

So, we made a decision: we would go on the cruise, Patty would postpone her hip replacement until 2019, and everything would hinge on whether my pancreatic work-up showed anything serious. We hadn't even booked flights yet.

It was an extraordinarily stressful time - too many variables, too many moving parts.

Then, out of nowhere, the phone rang.

On Friday, September 7th, Maria called back. Two extra surgical days had been added to the schedule. Eight hips would be done. Patty could have one of the slots — Friday, September 14th — if she could attend pre-op on Tuesday the 11th.

September 14th was the **last possible day** she could have surgery and still be allowed to fly ninety days later.

We didn't hesitate.

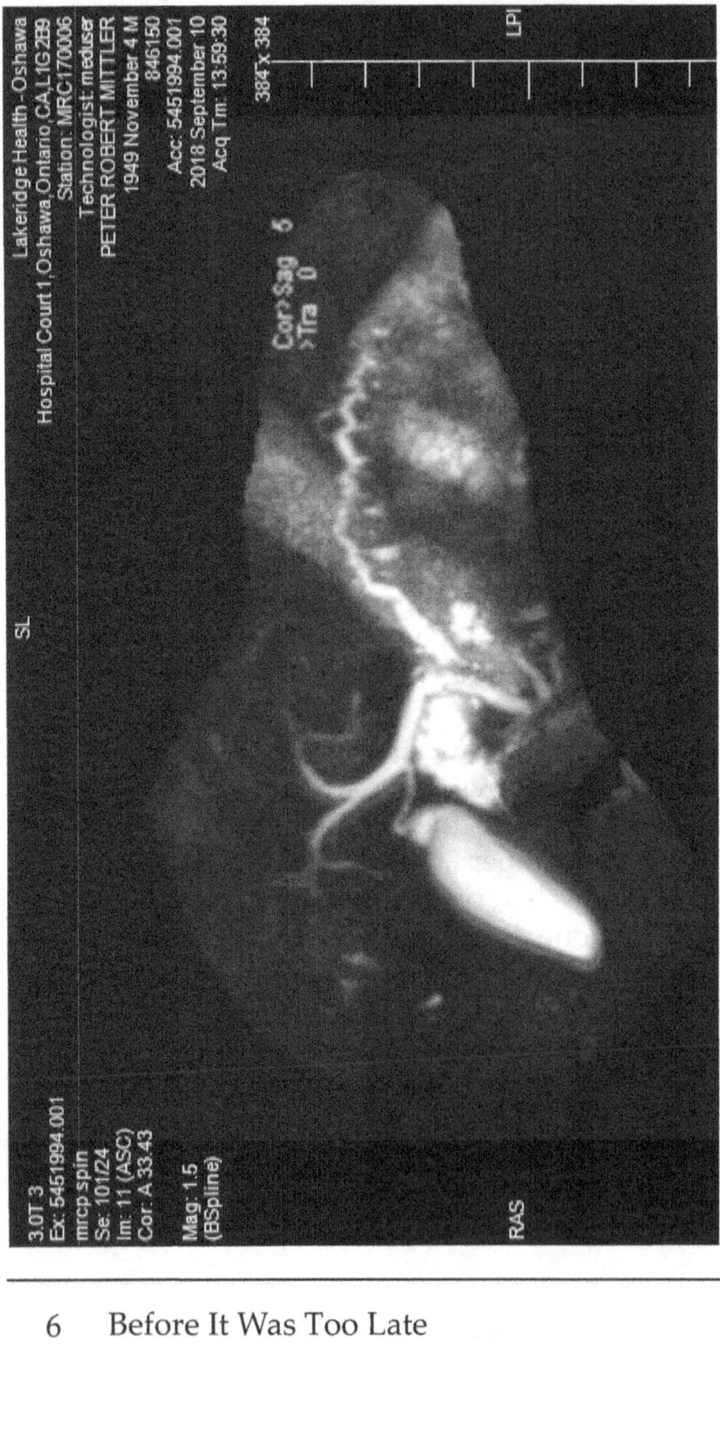

Photo 1: My diseased pancreas showing the dilated and circuitous duct.

Chapter 4: The Devlin Referral

September 24, 2018 — Patty's birthday.

Dr. Tim Devlin was looking at my MRI on his screen [Photo 1] when he said, "I have never seen anything like this in all my years of gastroenterology."

That got my attention."I'm sending you to my colleague, Dr. Gary May, at St. Michael's Hospital," he said. He is the best endoscopic gastroenterologist in the country. "And I'm marking this urgent."

On most days, there's no way to speed up the Ontario medical system. On this occasion, every doctor involved understood two things:

First, there was an emerging and serious pancreatic problem that needed immediate evaluation.

Secondly, if this turned out to be pancreatic cancer, the cruise might be the last time we were all together.

They understood that mattered.

Within weeks, I was booked for an endoscopic ultrasound. Dr. May promised pathology results within a week.

He managed to speed it up. Two days later, he called.

"Enjoy your cruise," he said. "You're cancer-free. I'll see you in six months."

The relief was enormous. For the moment, the shadow had lifted.

We went: Christmas on Majestic Princess sailing through New Zealand and Australia. It was wonderful. Grandson Ewan wrote a poem which I turned into a song. After the cruise Patty and I proceeded to Perth for our normal 'Canadian winter' stay. It wasn't life-threatening, so we put it aside.

But out of sight was not out of mind.

Chapter 5: Choice To Make

May 2020

Two years later — after three more episodes of pancreatitis — I was back in Dr. Gary May's office.

On paper, nothing dramatic had changed. There was still no definitive cancer. No metastatic disease. No single scan that screamed emergency.

But everything had changed.

Three more bouts of pancreatitis had left me weaker, more cautious, and increasingly aware that this problem wasn't going away. Imaging showed a pancreatic duct that was larger and more distorted than before. Cysts were multiplying. Inflammation was becoming the rule rather than the exception.

This time Dr. May didn't begin with reassurance.

He began with clarity.

"You have a choice," he said.

That's never as comforting as it sounds.

"Which is?"

"Sunnybrook or St. Joseph's. You need a total pancreatectomy."

"And if I do neither?"

He paused for a moment before answering.

"Then sometime around December," he said quietly, "we'll likely be having a conversation about palliative care."

That sentence landed exactly the way it was meant to.

I asked about alternatives — a Whipple procedure, a partial resection, anything that didn't involve removing the entire pancreas.

"No," he said. "Your pancreas is too diseased for that. The duct is massively dilated. The structure is abnormal throughout. This isn't localised — it's diffuse."

I asked about islet cell transplantation — moving insulin-producing cells to the liver to soften the blow of diabetes.

"At your age you are not a candidate," he said. "And even if you were, success rates are low."

Then he explained the part that mattered most.

Right now, I didn't have invasive cancer. But statistically the odds of developing it were very high. And once it appeared — once it metastasised — pancreatic surgery would no longer be an option.

This wasn't about treating cancer.
It was about preventing incurable cancer.
I didn't hesitate.

"Sunnybrook," I said.

And that was when everything truly began.

When he referred me to Sunnybrook Hospital, things began to move quickly.

At Sunnybrook, my case was reviewed by a multidisciplinary team — surgeons, radiologists, gastroenterologists, endocrinologists. Every scan going back years was pulled and re-examined. Patterns emerged that hadn't been obvious in isolation.

The main pancreatic duct had gone from mildly dilated to massively enlarged. The surrounding tissue showed changes that blurred the line between inflammation and early malignancy. Blood vessels were being affected. The portal vein, in particular, was at risk.

The conclusion was unanimous, and they concurred with Dr. May, a total pancreatectomy.

I met on the phone with Dr. Paul Karanicolas, the surgeon who would oversee the plan. He was direct, thorough, and unsentimental. He explained the operation in detail — not just what would be removed, but what life would look like afterward.

I would become an insulin-dependent diabetic overnight. Not the kind managed with pills or long buffers. The brittle kind. The kind where mistakes have consequences.

I would need pancreatic enzyme replacement for life. My diet would change. My margins would narrow.

Then he explained the risks: Bleeding. Infection. Anastomotic leaks. Vascular involvement. Death.

He quoted an in-hospital mortality risk of around three percent. I appreciated the honesty.

What mattered more to me was what would happen if I didn't do it.

We talked about timing. About waiting. About how inflammation could make surgery impossible if it progressed too far. About how cancer, if it appeared, would close the window entirely.

I asked for time to think.

I didn't need much.

When I agreed to proceed, the process accelerated.

Endocrinology was brought in early to prepare me for life without a pancreas. Diabetes education started before surgery — not after. Vaccinations were arranged in anticipation of losing my spleen.

This wasn't reactive medicine.

This was deliberate, planned, and purposeful.

The operating room was booked. Extra time was allocated. Backup plans were made.

The surgery was scheduled for July 22, 2020. COVID-19 was in full swing, and I still have the hospital admin sticker — the access pass — from that date on my CPAP machine.

I walked into Sunnybrook knowing exactly what I was giving up — and why.

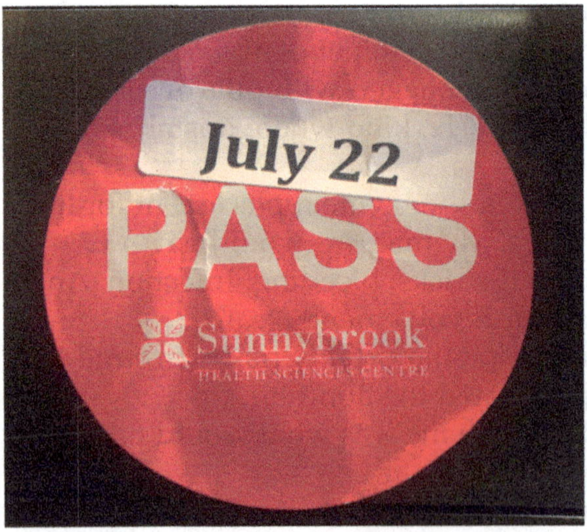

Photo 2: My 'COVID-19' pass to Sunnybrook Hospital. July 22, 2020.
This was the day I became a 'brittle diabetic'

The hardest part wasn't the fear of surgery.

It was accepting that waiting — doing nothing — was the most dangerous option of all.

Chapter 6: Surgery, Then That Fateful Hour

July 2020

At about 7 a.m. I was dropped at the hospital. I did my COVID-19 screening, got my pass and checked in.

The surgery lasted far longer than planned.

What was supposed to take about four hours stretched to seven. The inflammation was worse than expected. The pancreas and spleen were stuck to everything they shouldn't have been. At one point, separating the spleen from the portal vein became impossible, and the decision was made to resect and reconstruct the vein rather than risk catastrophic bleeding.

When it was over, I no longer had a pancreas.

Or a spleen.

Or a gallbladder.

Part of my stomach was gone, along with a section of my duodenum.

My bile duct had been rerouted.

Blood had been replaced.

Anatomy had been rearranged.

But the cancer everyone feared still wasn't there.

I woke up in recovery groggy, sore, and alive.

That felt like success.

The next day was difficult but manageable. Pain was controlled. Nurses were attentive. Endocrinology was already involved, guiding the transition to insulin. It was complicated, but it was orderly. There was a plan.

Then, on the second day after surgery, something shifted.

The second drama began

It wasn't dramatic at first. Just a feeling that something wasn't right. Discomfort. Shortness of breath. A vague sense of pressure that didn't fit neatly into the "post-operative pain" box.

Then the pain moved into my chest. And down my left arm.

The room changed quickly after that.

Monitors started to alarm. Blood pressure dropped. Faces appeared where there hadn't been faces before. Someone said, "rapid response." Someone else said, "ECG changes."

I didn't know it yet, but I was having a major heart attack.

At first, cardiology prepared to take me to the Cath lab. A stent seemed like the obvious solution. But then the blood work came back. My haemoglobin had significantly dropped. I was bleeding somewhere, or at least my body was behaving as if I were.

Taking me to the Cath lab now would likely kill me.

Everything stopped. And then everything moved again — in a different direction.

I was transferred to the cardiac intensive care unit. Fluids. Blood. Pressers. Endless assessments. The surgical team, the cardiology team, critical care — all of them now working the same problem from different angles.

At some point, Patty was called and told to come to the hospital.

That's a call no one ever wants their spouse to receive.

I didn't feel panic. What I felt instead was clarity.

The cath lab tried a stent but it made me unstable. I later understood that stents were not going to work for me. For reasons that were still unfolding, my body couldn't tolerate them. I also understood that if I survived this moment, the next step would not be easy.

When the cardiologist explained that my chances of surviving bypass surgery under these conditions were around twenty-five percent, I listened carefully.

While Patty was attending to me at the hospital, Matthew flew from Calgary to Toronto, even though he couldn't visit me in hospital because of COVID-19. Knowing he was there mattered. He arrived at the house while his mom was with me at Sunnybrook. Poor guy could not figure out how to turn on the lights since I had them all on Apple Home and voice commands.

My recollection of how it unfolded

A few days after the heart attack, once the immediate crisis had settled into something like stability, the Chief of cardiac surgery came to see me.

He didn't come alone.

He arrived with a small group — interns, residents, fellows — the next generation. This wasn't a casual visit. This was a teaching round.

He stood at the foot of the bed, reviewed the chart, and then spoke plainly.

He explained that I had suffered a major myocardial infarction. That my heart function was significantly compromised. That I was, by any reasonable measure, a very high-risk surgical candidate.

Then he said the number.

"If we attempt bypass surgery," he said, "your chance of survival is about twenty-five percent."

There was no drama in his voice. No softening of the edges. Just facts.

He went on to explain that a stent would normally be the preferred option — less invasive, faster recovery — but in my case it simply wasn't viable. My body hadn't tolerated it. The bleeding risk was too great. The anatomy too complex.

So, he laid out the reality.

We could try medical management and hope.

Or we could attempt the bypass and accept the odds.

I listened carefully. I wasn't shocked. By that point, numbers like that had stopped feeling abstract. They were just information.

Unbeknownst to me, my heart had grown its own emergency bypass—collateral vessels that rerouted blood around a dangerous blockage. According to my doctors, that detour probably kept me alive.

When he finished, I told him I didn't want them to attempt another stent. He looked slightly surprised.

I said something that had been clear to me since the moment things went sideways.

I related that when I was in CCU there was a photo in the ceiling light of a forest canopy, and I felt the comforting presence of an external calm. I could see a man's face in the photo.

And I heard a voice say, 'I am not finished with you yet, go back.' (I later used this image on the album cover my published song 'Joyous Moments").

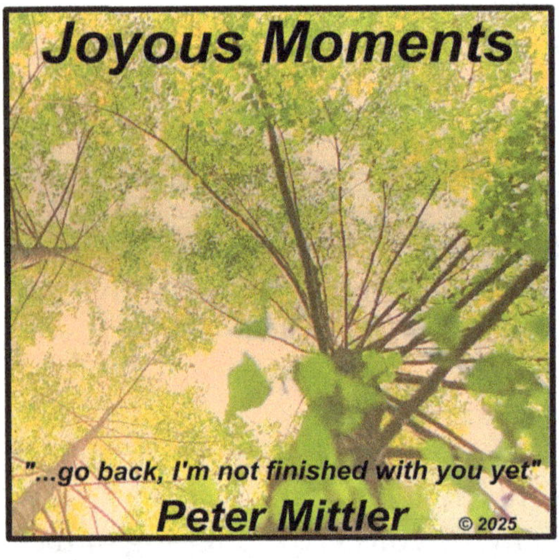

Photo 3: The significant ceiling light photo

When I woke up from that experience Patty was at my bedside. They had called her to come and see me.

"I believe one of two things will happen," I said. "Either I will die on the table and I will go to heaven — or I will survive because there is still something I am meant to do. I don't know what that is yet, but I'm certain I'm not finished."

The room went quiet.

He didn't challenge me. He didn't debate theology. He didn't try to correct my thinking.

Instead, he looked at me for a long moment, then turned slightly toward the trainees behind him.

"I have never," he said, "met a patient with such a strong survivor's attitude."

Then he looked back at me.

"If you want the bypass," he said, "we will design a plan to get you as strong as possible and we will do it."

That was the moment the conversation changed. From *if* to *how*.

From risk assessment to preparation.

From waiting to planning.

They left shortly after, and the unit settled back into its usual rhythm. Monitors. Medications. Nurses moving quietly in and out.

But something ha shifted.

For the first time since the heart attack, I wasn't just being managed.

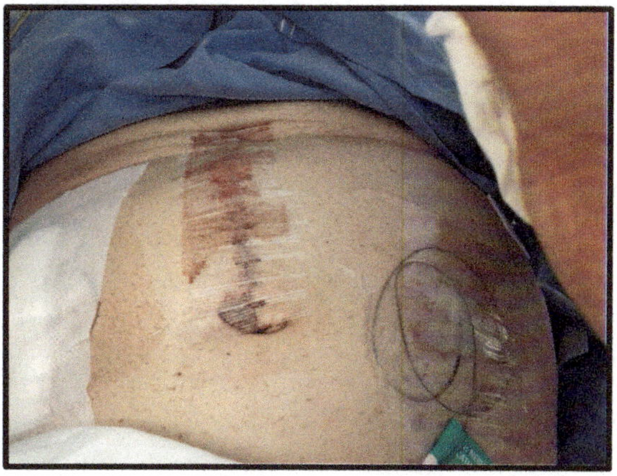

Photo 4: July 24, 2020 48 hours after the Pancreatectomy

I was being partnered with.

I spent the next ten days in the cardiac ICU while they stabilised me and figured out how to proceed. There were setbacks. I was moved to the recovery ward. At one point, while sitting on my walker, I fainted and ended up on the floor with the walker on top of me. That collapse would set off one of the most chaotic nights of my stay — a story I'll return to shortly.

Eventually, I was transferred out of ICU and into recovery again, this time to the Schulich Heart Institute — weaker now, thinner, diabetic, and very aware of how close the edge I had been.

Chapter 7: The Mad Dash

It was Tuesday, July 28 - I believe

I was using my walker in a four-person ward when I had a syncope event. I fainted without warning and fell off the walker I had been sitting on. It tipped over and landed on top of me, pinning me partially under the bed. At the time, I didn't understand what had happened or why. It would have been almost funny if it hadn't been so dangerous.

They got me back onto a bed, and that's when the decision was made to return me to the Cardiac Care Unit.

The nurse who attended me knelt beside the bed and spoke calmly and directly.

"Mr. Mittler," she said, "in order to move you back to CCU, we have to take you down an elevator. For that, we need to put paddles on you. And hospital protocol requires that I call a Code Blue so I can access the crash cart. This Code Blue is administrative only. I don't want you to panic when the ward suddenly fills with people."

I told her I understood.

Then she called the Code Blue.

Within seconds, it felt as though the entire hospital had descended on me. My gown was ripped open, paddles were placed on my chest, and I was transferred onto a mobile bed.

The noise, the urgency, the sheer number of people—it was overwhelming.

Outside, a massive thunderstorm was raging. I could hear it. The lights flickered.

As we moved rapidly down the hallway, the power went out.

The hospital shifted to emergency mode. I distinctly heard someone call out, "Does anyone have the key for the elevator?" The regular elevators were down. They needed the emergency one.

I also became acutely aware that my hospital gown was flapping open and that my dignity was being sacrificed to the moment. Somewhere in that chaos, a strange thought crossed my mind: *This feels like I'm on the set of Grey's Anatomy.*

They finally got me into a very small emergency elevator—possibly running on generator power by now. One person stood at my head, another at the foot of the bed. The rest of the team took the stairs, running.

Down we went.

They met us at the bottom, rushed me through another set of elevators, and delivered me into CCU.

And then something extraordinary happened.

Out of forty-three possible rooms, they took me into the same room I had been in before. The same room! The same bed. And above me, the same image of a forest canopy—the one that had been there during my earlier stay, when I had experienced something deeply personal and profound.

Seeing it again settled me.

In that moment, despite the chaos, the storm, the alarms, and the fear, I felt an unexpected calm. As if my future—whatever it might hold—was safe, guided, and held by something larger than myself.

After stabilisation in CCU, I was transferred to the Schulich Heart Institute — a move that would repeat itself more than once. It was there that I began to recover slowly, walk the halls and reflect on what just hit me.

Chapter 8: Ten Days Became Thirty

I ended up back in the Schulich Heart Institute, where I would spend the next month rebuilding strength and waiting for the next step.

Days stopped feeling like days. Nights were indistinguishable from mornings. Everything was measured in numbers — blood pressure, heart rate, oxygen saturation, glucose levels — and in short conversations that carried enormous weight.

I had survived the pancreatic surgery.

I had survived the heart attack.

I had dodged pancreatic cancer.

But now I was in a kind of medical limbo.

Before bypass could even be attempted, my rhythm had to be stabilised.

The cardiology team was trying to understand what

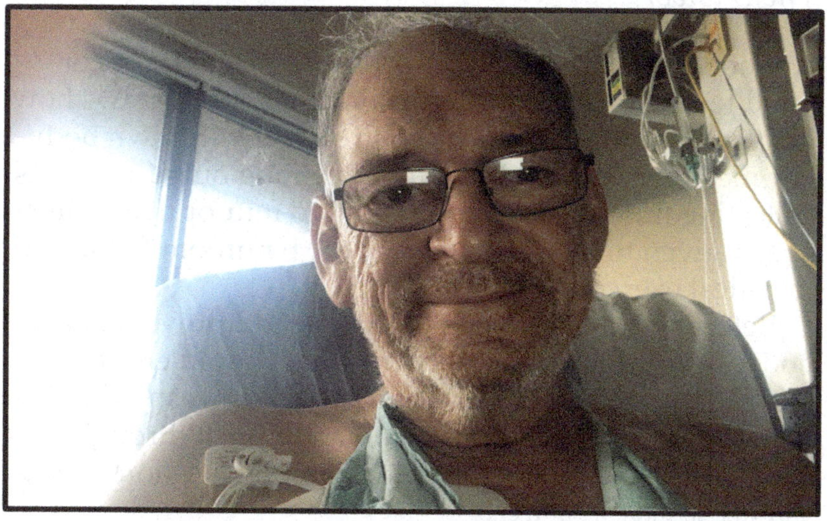

Photo 5: August 3, 2020. Ten days after Pancreatectomy and eight days after the heart attack

had happened and what could safely be done next. A stent, under normal circumstances, would have been the obvious solution. In my case, it wasn't. My body simply couldn't tolerate it. The risk of bleeding was too high, and the anatomy — altered by major abdominal surgery — complicated everything.

So, they waited. And watched. And stabilised.

I was weak. I had lost blood. I was learning, in real time, what it meant to live without a pancreas. Blood sugar swings came quickly and without warning. There was no buffer anymore. Every decision mattered.

COVID-19 restrictions were still in place, but Sunnybrook did what it could. Patty was not allowed to be there. The staff understood that this wasn't just a medical crisis — it was a human one.

The days stretched on. I got bored.

The Shower

Anyone who has spent a long stretch in hospital—confined to a bed and reduced to sponge baths—knows how discouraging it feels to lose control over your own body. For me, it was worse. I had tubes coming out of me, bags collecting fluid, and I was tethered to four or five IV lines at any given time. Even going to the bathroom felt like a logistical exercise.

Before I could go home, they insisted I prove that my body could function on its own—that I could empty my bladder and bowels without assistance. It wasn't dignified, but it was necessary, and I had to push through it.

Then one day, a nurse asked a simple question: *Would you like to have a shower?*

They disconnected what they could, left the IV lines in place, and helped me into the bathroom. Standing under running water, feeling clean again, felt almost miraculous. For a few minutes, I wasn't a patient or a problem to be managed. I was just a person.

That shower remains one of the most wonderful experiences I had in the hospital. Not because it was extraordinary, but because it reminded me of who I still was.

CABG or not?

Eventually, the cardiology team sat down with me and laid it out plainly. If I wanted the best chance at meaningful recovery, I would need a double CABG surgery. (Coronary Arterial Bypass Graft). Not immediately — my body wasn't ready — but soon. Very soon.

I listened carefully. They explained that they could only do a double bypass because there was a lot of dead heart tissue and feeding new blood into dead tissue wasn't going to revive it. Thus forget about a 'triple' or a 'quad' bypass.

I understood the risks. I had already been told that my odds were not good. Twenty-five percent was the number that kept coming up. Not encouraging. Not comforting.

But I also understood something else.

I had already come this far by earlier choosing the harder option. Waiting had never served me well. Acting — thoughtfully, deliberately — had.

So, I said yes to the double CABG.

I chose the higher risk option.

Again.

Those ten days in the CCU felt longer than the weeks I had spent preparing for surgery. They were filled with uncertainty, discomfort, and a constant low-level awareness that things could still go wrong.

But slowly, almost imperceptibly, they didn't.

My numbers stabilised. My strength began to return in small increments. The plan took shape.

When I was finally transferred out of the CCU and back into a recovery ward, it felt like crossing a quiet but important threshold.

I wasn't finished; I was still in the game!

Waiting for the Arrhythmia Lab

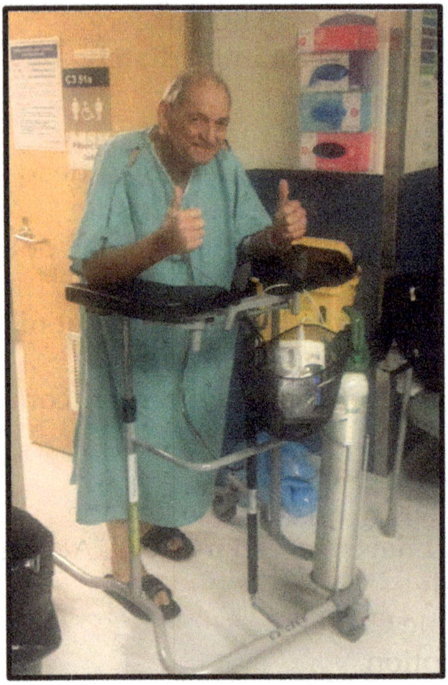

Photo 6: Doing the Dhama walk!

Before I could have bypass surgery, the team decided I needed to go home for about a month with a pacemaker in place. That meant one thing: I had to wait for a slot in the arrhythmia lab. They kept telling me it was coming—soon—but no one could say exactly when.

Two weeks into my stay in the Schulich Heart Institute, I was getting noticeably stronger. Peter Dhama called me every day, and I was walking the floors of the Schulich Cardiac Institute, feeling my strength return step by step. At that point, all I really wanted was to go home. The waiting was harder than the recovery.

To pass the time—and probably to stay sane—I wrote

four or five songs on my guitar during those days. Still, my patience was wearing thin.

Every morning I'd be told, ***Tomorrow we'll put the pacemaker in.*** And every day, right around noon, someone would arrive with my lunch and the same update: Not today. Someone else is more emergent.

It happened again and again. I was bumped down the list so often that I finally wrote a song called "Hurry up and Wait: Bumped Again" It was gallows humour, but it helped.

Eventually, the day did come. A Boston Scientific pacemaker was implanted, and not long after that, I was discharged. Walking out of the hospital and heading home felt like a victory—hard-earned, delayed, but deeply satisfying.

Dark Horse

One day, while I was recovering I got an unexpected call from Peter Dhama, a friend in the MG Car Club of Toronto. Peter subsequently called me every day to check in and see how I was doing.

On this day, he asked how many times the nurses had asked me to walk around the station. I told him they wanted me to do two laps sometime that day.

He said, "How many have you done?"

I said, "None."

Without missing a beat, he said, "Get off your

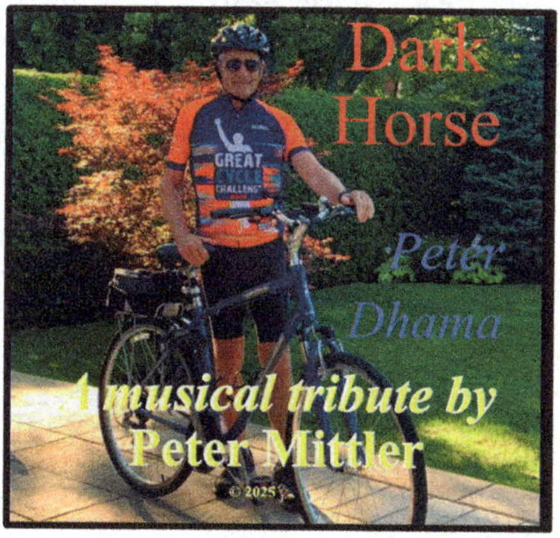

Photo 7: Peter Dhama, encourager

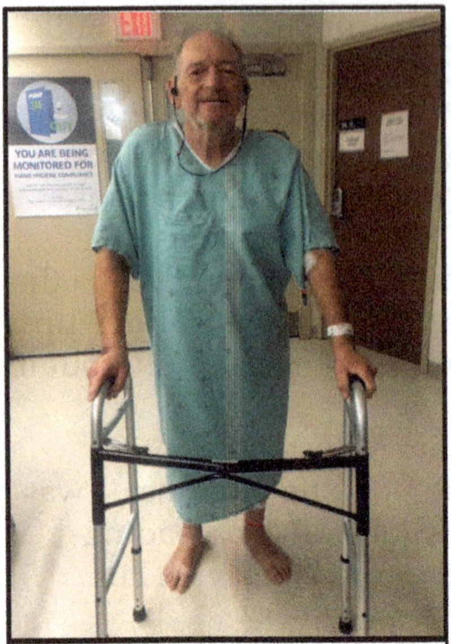

Photo 8: Finally shedding the IV's and doing more Dhama lap

fucking ass and go do one. I'll call you back later," and he hung up.

About four hours later, he rang again.

"Well," he said, "did you do one?"

"Yes."

"How long did it take?"

"About an hour."

"Good," he said. "Let's have a chat."

We talked about nothing important at all — but everything he said was encouraging. Just before he hung up, he told me to go and do another lap.

Later that night, around nine o'clock, he called again.

"Did you do another one?"

"Yes."

"Good," he said. "I'll call you tomorrow."

Peter was instrumental in pushing me through my recovery when my body didn't want to cooperate. He believed in me when I wasn't sure I could. For that, I owe him more than I can say.

I later wrote a song about him — *Dark Horse*.

FaceTime Calls with Alyssa

Our daughter, Alyssa, lives in Perth, Australia. She is a paediatric cardiac CCU nurse—at least she was at the time. Because she worked night shifts, the timing aligned in an extraordinary way: when the doctors came around on rounds at Sunnybrook, it was often three o'clock in the afternoon for us and three o'clock in the morning for her.

On many occasions, Alyssa would FaceTime into my iPad and join the doctors during rounds to discuss my care. The Sunnybrook staff were most receptive to this process as well. Alyssa also spent a great deal of time reading the doctors' notes in the Sunnybrook Health Records system, using my login, so she had a clear and current understanding of what was being proposed and what was actually being done.

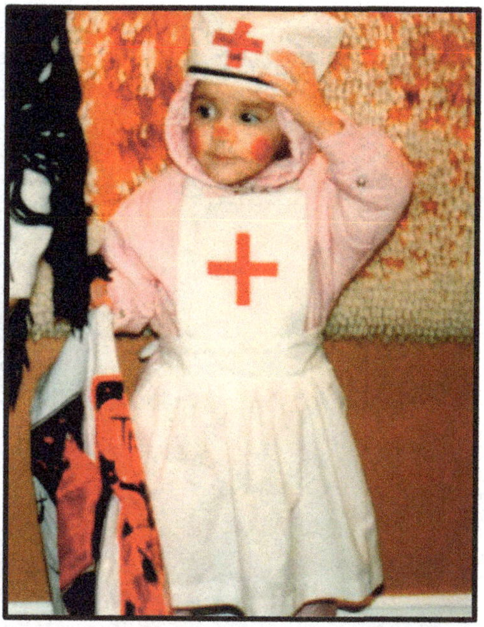

Photo 9: Alyssa the nurse

The beauty of this was that she could then interpret everything for me—translating complex medical language into words I could understand. It was deeply comforting to have a family member who was also a medical professional watching over my care, validating what the doctors were doing, and explaining it to me in real time.

What I didn't fully grasp then—but Alyssa did—was just how close I came to losing my life. She understood the seriousness of what was happening in a way I could not. She never told me how dire things truly were, but I now know that she knew. And somehow, that makes her quiet presence during those FaceTime calls even more profound.

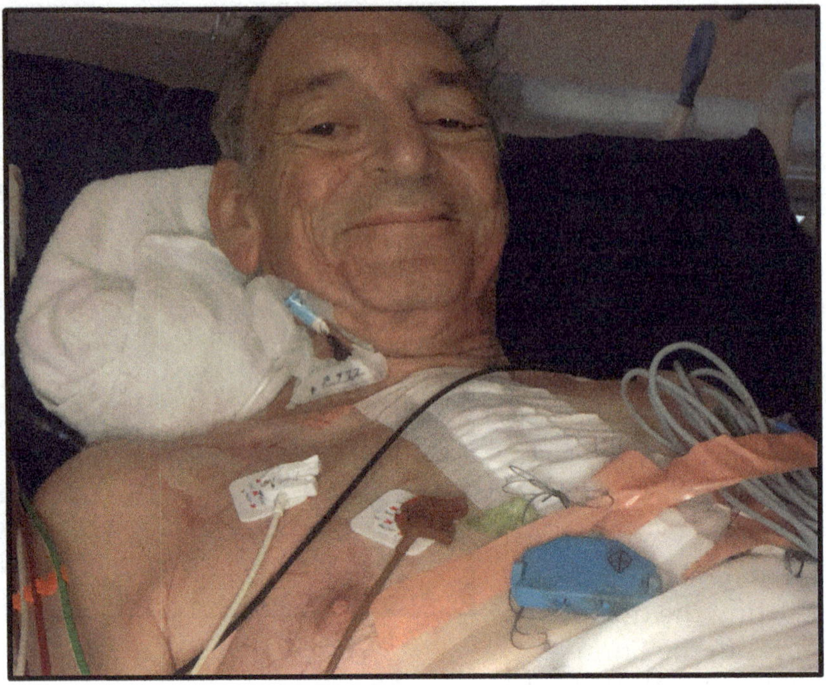

Photo 10 Early in cardiac recovery. Happy to be alive

The Creon Fiasco

When you become a Type 3C diabetic because your pancreas has been surgically removed, the problem isn't just insulin. That part is obvious enough. What is less obvious—at least to many people—is that you also lose the pancreatic enzymes that make digestion possible: protease, lactase, and amylase. Without them, food passes through the body largely unprocessed, offering little nourishment no matter how much you eat. Check out Appendix C for a Type 1/2/3 comparison.

To replace that missing enzyme suite, you must take Creon—C-R-E-O-N. Creon is a capsule derived from porcine pancreas and is a well-established substitute for the enzymes lost after a pancreatectomy. For me, the regimen was simple and non-negotiable: two capsules before every meal and one before every snack. Eight a day. Period.

The crucial word there is *before*.

Creon must be taken prior to eating so that the enzymes are present when food enters the stomach. Taken afterward, it is largely ineffective. The enzymes sit uselessly on top of the meal, unable to do the work they are designed to do. Timing is everything.

Unfortunately, many of the nurses in the CCU and the Schulich Heart Institute were unfamiliar with this distinction. Habitually, they would bring my prescribed dose of Creon *after* I had finished eating. From a nursing workflow perspective, it probably made sense. From a physiological perspective, it made none at all.

After this happened repeatedly, I decided to take matters into my own hands. I asked that my Creon be brought in from home, and I began self-dosing—taking it correctly, before meals, when it could actually do its job.

That arrangement worked well until one particular encounter.

One day, a nurse came to me after a meal and insisted that I take the Creon she had brought. I explained that I had already taken my dose before eating. She was not satisfied. When I declined to take another dose unnecessarily, she became indignant and demanded that I swallow it.

I asked her to place the capsule in my hand so that I could replace the one I had taken from my own supply—ensuring I would still have the correct number available for the next meal. That suggestion did not go over well.

Instead, she escalated the situation by calling the head nurse.

I then found myself explaining—again—that Creon is a pancreatic enzyme replacement that must be taken *before* meals, not after. I explained that I was perfectly capable of managing this medication myself, and that I understood my condition and its requirements intimately.

None of this seemed to satisfy her. In the end, simply to keep the peace, I took the additional Creon she insisted upon—despite knowing it served no useful purpose at that point.

Fortunately, that was the only time the issue escalated to that level. Afterward, the nursing staff became more familiar with my situation and accepted that I knew what I was doing. The problem did not recur.

But the episode stayed with me.

It was a small incident in the grand scheme of things—no alarms, no codes, no dramatic interventions. Yet it highlighted something important: survival does not end with surgery. It depends just as much on knowledge, timing, and communication. And sometimes, the patient is the person in the room who understands those things best.

Getting the Insulin Dose Right

I thought getting the insulin dose right would be straightforward. After all, this was a major teaching hospital, and insulin management is something hospitals deal with every day. What I underestimated was how different things become when the pancreas is gone entirely.

Without a pancreas, insulin isn't being *supplemented*—it's being *replaced*. There is no baseline, no background production, no physiological safety net. Every unit matters. Too little, and blood sugars climb relentlessly. Too much, and you risk a hypoglycaemic crash. It's a narrow path, and it takes time, observation, and adjustment to find the right balance.

In practice, they struggled with it.

My blood glucose readings swung more than anyone seemed comfortable admitting. Doses were adjusted, then adjusted again, sometimes reacting to the last number rather than the overall pattern. What worked one day didn't necessarily work the next. Meals, stress, recovery, inactivity, and digestion—all of it played a role, and not always in predictable ways.

Part of the difficulty was that I wasn't a typical diabetic patient. I wasn't Type 1. I wasn't Type 2. I was Type 3C—diabetic because my pancreas had been surgically removed. That distinction matters, but it's not one many clinicians deal with often, especially outside endocrinology.

There was no negligence here, just unfamiliarity. Still, living inside those fluctuating numbers was unsettling. I could feel when things were off—fatigue, fogginess, a strange internal unease that didn't show up clearly on a monitor. And yet, from the outside, it all looked like routine insulin management.

Over time, things improved. Patterns emerged. Doses became more stable. But it was far from the simple, solved problem I had assumed it would be.

What I learned—again—was that surviving a complex surgery means entering a long period where medicine is as much trial and adjustment as it is protocol. And when your body no longer behaves like the textbook example, even well-intentioned systems can struggle to keep up.

I was placed on a daily dose of Lantus, a long-acting basal insulin, and for meals they used a standard bolus of short-acting insulin—typically five to seven units of NovoRapid. On paper, this seemed to work reasonably well. My numbers were not wildly out of range, and there was at least a sense that we were heading in the right direction.

Still, getting the dose right proved elusive.

The young endocrinology registrar assigned to my care struggled with the unpredictability of my blood sugars. I don't blame her. I don't think she had ever managed a patient who had no pancreas at all. Without endogenous insulin, glucagon, or any buffering response, my glucose levels could shift quickly and without warning. What looked like inconsistency was really physiology operating without its usual safeguards.

Complicating matters further was how my blood glucose was being measured.

By that point, I had managed to obtain a Freestyle Libre continuous glucose monitor. I trusted it. It gave me trend data, warnings, and a sense of direction—whether my sugars were rising, falling, or holding steady. The hospital, however, trusted finger-stick testing. Hospital protocol required it. And so, despite wearing a CGM, I continued to endure frequent finger pricks.

Invariably, the results were very close.

The irony did not escape me.

What made the situation more challenging was that some of the cardiac nurses had little experience performing finger-stick glucose tests. A few did not fully appreciate the importance of *when* the test was done. Timing matters. Blood glucose must be measured *before* insulin is administered, not afterward. Doing it the other way around renders the information largely meaningless.

More than once, I found myself explaining this—gently, but firmly. In a strange reversal of roles, I became, in a sense, an educator. I was teaching members of the cardiac care team how to manage a diabetic patient, even as I lay in a hospital bed recovering from major surgery.

It wasn't anyone's fault. It was a mismatch between specialisation and circumstance. But it reinforced a lesson

I kept learning throughout my recovery: when your condition falls outside the norm, you sometimes become the most knowledgeable person in the room about your own care.

By this point, my care had become a constant exercise in measurement, adjustment, and timing. Enzymes, insulin, glucose readings—everything revolved around numbers. But what none of those numbers could fully capture was how it actually felt to live inside a body without its usual safeguards.

Living Between the Numbers

Blood glucose management, I learned, is not just about numbers. It is about how those numbers feel.

There were moments when my readings looked acceptable, even reassuring, yet my body told a different story. Like a heaviness behind the eyes; a mental fog that made conversation feel like work; subtle internal unease that didn't register on any chart. At other times, the numbers dipped or climbed quickly, and I felt it before anyone else noticed.

Without a pancreas, there is no buffering system—no gentle correction happening quietly in the background. Every fluctuation is experienced directly. You live between readings, aware that what matters most is not the number itself but the direction it is heading and how fast it is moving.

That was where the CGM helped most. It didn't just report data; it told a story. It showed trends, momentum, and risk. A single finger-stick reading was a snapshot. The CGM was a narrative. And when you are living inside that narrative, you learn to listen to your body as carefully as you can.

Protocol vs Physiology

Hospitals run on protocols, and for good reason. Protocols create safety, consistency, and accountability. But protocols are designed for typical cases, and not all patients are typical.

My physiology had been fundamentally altered. I no longer fit neatly into any standard category. I wasn't a Type 1 diabetic, and I certainly wasn't Type 2. I was a surgical outlier—Type 3C—living without the organs that usually smooth out metabolic chaos.

Yet the protocols didn't always bend easily. Finger-stick testing was required, even when a CGM was providing accurate, real-time data. Insulin dosing followed standard ranges, even when my responses fell outside predictable patterns. Timing rules were applied uniformly, even when timing was just the thing that needed individualisation.

This wasn't about incompetence or indifference. It was about systems encountering edge cases. And edge cases expose the limits of even the best-designed rules.

What saved me, more often than not, was conversation—explaining, asking, insisting when necessary. Care improved when protocol made room for physiology instead of trying to override it.

Advocacy as Survival

Looking back, one of the most important skills I developed during my recovery was not medical at all. It was advocacy.

I learned to speak up—sometimes gently, sometimes firmly. I learned when to accept guidance and when to question it. I learned that being a "good patient" does not mean being a silent one. It means being engaged,

Chorus from Angels in Blue

Nurses are angels out on the floor,
Serving you gladly nothing's a chore,
When you're in pain and very perturbed,
Comforting words from a nurse can be heard.

---

informed, and willing to participate actively in your own care.

This was not always comfortable. Hospitals are hierarchical places. Roles are clearly defined. But illness collapses those hierarchies in subtle ways. When you are living inside an altered body, you become an expert in that body whether you want to or not.

In my case, advocacy was not about confrontation. It was about collaboration. It was about ensuring that timing, dosing, and understanding aligned with reality rather than assumption.

Survival, I came to realise, does not depend solely on the brilliance of surgeons or the sophistication of machines. It also depends on attention, communication, and the courage to say, "This doesn't feel right," even when everything appears to be under control.

Once the immediate medical crises eased, something else began to surface—an awareness that survival is not sustained by protocols alone. Beyond numbers, machines, and carefully managed doses, there were moments when what mattered most was human presence. Sometimes that presence arrived quietly. And sometimes it arrived loudly, at exactly the moment it was needed.

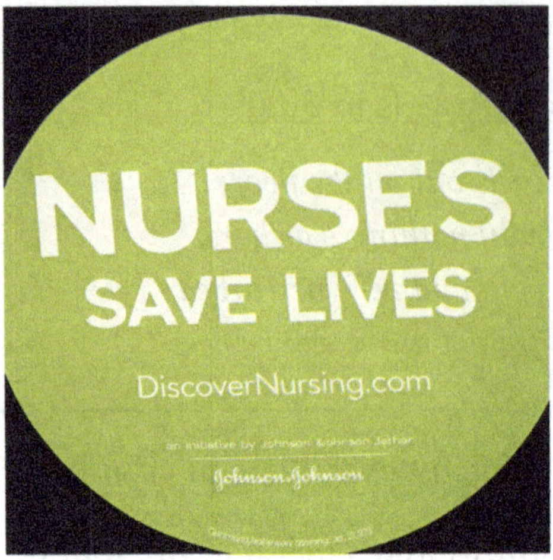

Photo 11 A poster at the nurses station

By this point, survival was no longer only about numbers and medication. It was about people.

The Salt Nurse

When I was in the Schulich Heart Institute, one of the things I missed having were little snacks. But I quickly found out that the gift shop down on the main floor would deliver up to my floor. So, I called them, ordered some snacks, paid with a credit card, and had them brought up.

It was great to have those snacks, which made me feel like I was less of a prisoner in my own room. I used them once in a while when I needed a feeling of crunch or a nosh.

But one day, a nurse came into my room, saw that, and, with a firm but compassionate tone, said to me, "Mr. Mittler, I want you to hear something very important. So many of the patients that I see in here can't lay off the salt. And the problem with eating those things is that water follows salt. You already have slight oedema in your legs, and we do not want to strain your kidneys by having you drink more water and retain water. And so I'm telling you right now to cut out those snacks and eat something that doesn't have salt in it, because you may end up on a dialysis machine on top of all of your pancreatectomy and cardiac issues. Do you want that? I don't think so. So lay off the salt."

Her words carried a sense of tough love, making it clear that she was looking out for my well-being. I knew she was right, and that moment left a lasting impression on me.

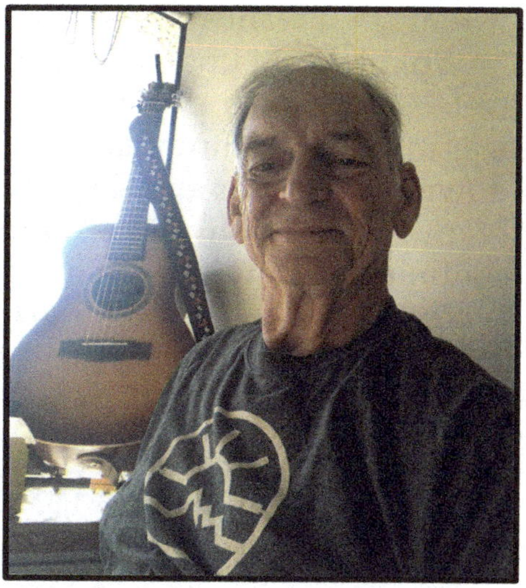

Photo 12: Musical therapy in recovery

The Screaming Angel

I was profoundly impressed by the nursing care I received throughout my time in the Schulich Heart Institute. From intake to the operating room, to recovery—twice over—the consistency, professionalism, and humanity of the nursing staff never wavered.

I was so moved by their presence and dedication that I later wrote a song called *Angels in Blue,* followed by *Echoes of Angels in Blue*. Both were written as tributes to the nurses who carried me through that period and are now available on Spotify and Apple Music.

One night, around 2:30 a.m., the quiet routine of the ward was shattered by a commotion in the room next door. A woman's voice rang out, raw and desperate, calling for an attendant. "I shat myself," she cried loudly and repeatedly. Sleep in hospital is elusive at the best of times—lights never fully dim, machines hum and beep incessantly, and alarms seem to exist in a permanent state of readiness. That night, the noise felt unbearable. Exhausted, sore, and short-tempered, my first reaction was anger. I wanted the screaming to stop.

What I didn't understand at first—what I could only feel—was that her pain wasn't only physical. There was fear in her voice, humiliation, and isolation. It carried down the corridor and sat heavily in the air. During one of my supervised walks around the ward, while her cries continued and no one seemed to be responding quickly enough, I asked a nearby nurse if I might go into her room to speak with her. They agreed on the strict condition that we remain two metres apart.

I entered with every intention of telling her—firmly—to settle down. But before I could say a word, she looked at me and asked, "Are you the one who's been playing music in the room next door?" I said that I was. She told me she had been listening, and that the songs helped her. She said they calmed her. I was completely disarmed.

Later, I asked the charge nurse why the common room at the end of the corridor was locked. There was nowhere for patients to gather, no shared space at all. The answer was simple: COVID-19 lockdown. No communal areas, no interaction. We were confined not only by illness, but by protocol. I remember pushing back, frustrated. If we had all been isolated in the hospital for weeks without visitors, how exactly were we supposed to infect one another? It made no sense—but rules were rules.

Still, after some discussion, they agreed to make an exception. My neighbouring room mate and I were escorted, masked and carefully distanced, into the common room. I sang for her there—ten feet apart—and recorded *Joyous Moments* during that session. The change in her was immediate. She settled. Her breathing slowed. Later, the nursing staff told me that the time we spent together made her easier to care for and reduced her distress significantly.

I'm not finished with you yet

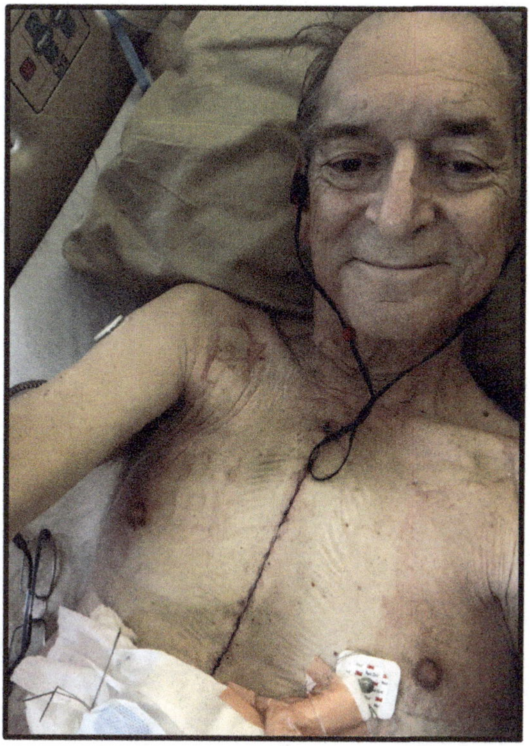

Photo 13: The lines came off but the scars remained

That moment marked a quiet turning point for me. For the first time after my surgeries, I realised that I still had something to give. Singing wasn't just helping others—it was helping me. It rebuilt lung capacity, gave structure to my days, and reminded me of who I was beyond the machines and the diagnoses. More than that, it planted a seed.

Four years later, that seed would grow into regular visits. Don Dowling, my playing partner and I, now perform volunteer concerts at aged-care facilities in Perth in a duo known as ***Hamersely Jam.*** We bring music to people who are shut in and struggling in ways both familiar and new.

What happened with my agitated neighbour showed me that recovery is not only about survival. It is also about rediscovering purpose.

In that locked ward, during COVID-19 lockdown, I found mine again.

Chapter 9: Learning How to Live Again

Late 2020 - 2021

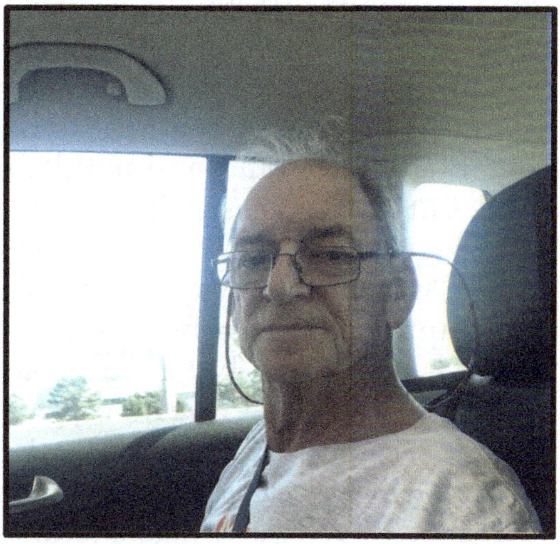

Photo 14: It felt like heaven to go home

Recovery after the bypass was different from everything that had come before.

What I was rebuilding now wasn't just physical strength, but a sense of who I still was.

This wasn't about surviving an acute crisis. It was about rebuilding a life that had been fundamentally altered.

I went home thinner, weaker, and carrying more medical equipment and medications than I ever imagined I would need. I was now living without a pancreas, without a spleen, and with a heart that had been through a major insult.

I was also a brittle diabetic.

There are no practice runs. No grace period. Mistakes show up quickly and demand immediate correction. I learned to pay attention to my body in ways I never had before — to patterns, to warning signs, to small changes that mattered more than they used to.

Endocrinology followed me closely. Education continued. Adjustments were constant. This was not a "set it and forget it" condition. It required engagement. Discipline. Respect.

One of the doctors once said, "Mr. Mittler, only five in fifteen million people in Ontario, in any one year, would survive what you went through. You are very lucky."

Some called it luck. I never did. I believe God was present through every step of that journey, working quietly through the doctors, nurses, and friends who chose to act when the moment mattered.

Four weeks after the first surgery, once I was stable enough, I went back in for the bypass. That operation, remarkably, went more smoothly. Recovery was still hard, but it was measurable — not a return to normal, but progress. Enough to move forward.

By October, there were signs that my heart function was improving. By early 2021, I was finding a rhythm again — a new one, but a workable one.

By May of 2022, I was doing well. Not in a dramatic way. Just steadily. Thoughtfully. Responsibly.

I was alive. I was active. I was present.

Looking back now, what stands out isn't just the skill of the surgeons or the sophistication of the medicine — though both were extraordinary. What stands out is how often the outcome hinged on timing, attention, and the willingness to act before certainty arrived.

Modern medicine saved my life.

People paid attention. People listened. People were willing to move quickly when the window was open.

I don't think of this story as one about illness. I think of it as a story about paying attention — and choosing not to wait until it's too late.

God always had "One More Move." In 2025, I even wrote a song with that title.

Chapter 10: Going Home

October 2020

Going home isn't an ending. It's a transition.

Discharge did not feel like release so much as responsibility. The hospital routines fell away all at once, along with the constant surveillance that had quietly held me together. At home, time slowed dramatically. The pacemaker monitored my rhythm, but stamina was fragile and unpredictable. Simple tasks carried weight. Everything took longer.

Patty stepped into a role she never asked for and never hesitated to assume. She became chief cook, medication manager, logistics coordinator, appointment tracker, and caregiver—often all before breakfast. She learned schedules, dosages, warning signs, and contingencies, quietly absorbing the load while making it look manageable. I could not have done this without her.

We still had the walker left over from Patty's hip surgeries. It became mine now. Patty and I began walking together, cautiously at first. Three houses. Then five. Then ten. Progress was measured in driveways and mailboxes, not kilometres. October unfolded around us as we moved—leaves turning colour, air cooling, neighbours pausing to watch and wave. Some offered words of encouragement. Others simply nodded, as if understanding this was work that needed no commentary.

Later in the day, I would sit on the deck with my guitar as the sun dropped lower in the sky. I played quietly—not performing, just occupying the space. Flying bugs were relentless. The maple tree beside the house shifted from green to deep red, one branch at a time. These moments mattered more than I expected. They marked continuity. I was still here to notice them.

My doctor, Larry Bacher, helped close one chapter and open another. He arranged for my care to transition closer to home, connecting me with a cardiologist, Dr. Yadegari, so recovery could continue without the burden of long travel or institutional distance. It felt like another small but important step toward normalcy.

Recovery was not dramatic. There were no sudden leaps forward, no cinematic milestones—only persistence. It was incremental—uneven, sometimes frustrating, always humbling. But it was real. Each small gain held. Each day added quietly to the next.

Going home did not restore the life I had before.

It allowed me to begin building the one that would follow.

A life my friend Jon Rosenthall did not get a chance to share.

Chapter 11: Resetting the Compass

Winter 2020–2021 – through 2022

During the winter of 2020–2021, creativity returned before strength. My body lagged behind, slow to trust itself again, but my mind had already begun to re-engage. I found myself drawn back to familiar anchors: the steady rhythm of the lathe, the discipline of shaping wood; the act of writing music, line by line, note by note. These were not grand gestures of recovery. They were small, deliberate acts of return.

I tired easily. Fatigue arrived without warning, and sleep became a necessity rather than a luxury. Progress was uneven, sometimes frustratingly so. But what never left me was resolve. The will to participate fully in life again remained intact, even when energy did not.

MG 2022

In 2020, during the uncertainty of COVID-19, it was far from obvious that a national MG convention would even be possible in 2022. Because of my upcoming surgery, I had stepped back from my role as chairman of the convention committee, just in case things did not go well and I could not continue.

But by late 2021, as confidence slowly rebuilt, I found myself ready to return. Carefully, and with intention, I asked to resume the role of Chairman for MG 2022. It was not about reclaiming a title or status. It felt more like stewardship — an opportunity to contribute, to serve, and to honour commitments while respecting the limits my body had recently imposed.

Leadership, I was learning, did not require force.

It required attention.

Recovery, however, rarely proceeds in a straight line.

Pacemaker Failure

One of the first things that happened after we emigrated to Perth was a visit to my new cardiologist.

He asked, "Were you using a cardiac monitor back in Ontario?"

"What's a cardiac monitor?" I replied.

He explained that it was a small device that sits beside your bed and communicates with your pacemaker by Wi-Fi, allowing the hospital or your cardiologist to monitor it remotely.

"That sounds wonderful," I said. "Unfortunately Sunnybrook Hospital doesn't do that. I have to go into the hospital every three to six months to have it checked."

He looked surprised.

"That's a bit antiquated."

Apparently Sunnybrook could remotely monitor Medtronic devices, but not Boston Scientific pacemakers like mine. I never did discover why. It was a small reminder that, as outstanding as Sunnybrook Hospital was in its surgical departments, some aspects of their monitoring systems had not yet caught up with the times.

One day in May 2022 I drove down to the Arrhythmia Clinic at Sunnybrook Hospital — a 42-kilometre trip each way through heavy Toronto traffic, plus tolls and parking. In other words, a costly and inconvenient journey just to have my Boston Scientific pacemaker checked.

Up to that point, every visit had been routine.

The technician placed a magnetic device over the pace-

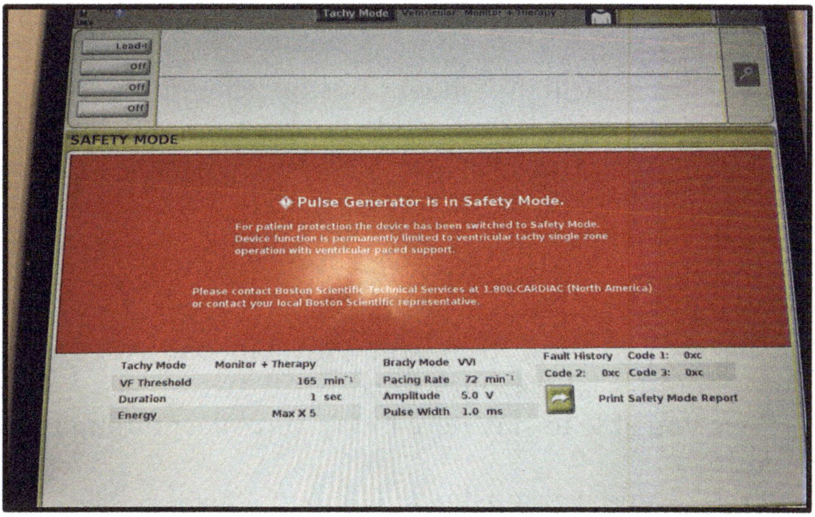

Photo 15 This is what the technician saw on her screen during the test of my pacemaker

maker to run diagnostics. As the system connected, she suddenly gasped and muttered under her breath.

"Oh shit."

I heard her.

"What do you mean 'oh shit'? That's my pacemaker."

She studied the screen.

"Mr. Mittler, something very strange is showing up here. Your pacemaker has gone into safety mode and it's pacing you at 72 beats per minute."

Trying to stay calm, I said, "Well, you've got remote access to it, don't you? Why don't you just reboot it?"

In my mind I was thinking about Windows computers — Ctrl-Alt-delete the problem and restart.

She shook her head.

"No. I can't do that. I have to get the Boston Scientific representative in here."

Sunnybrook used several different pacemaker systems — Boston Scientific, Medtronic, and another whose name escapes me — and the companies rotated support coverage every few days.

By sheer coincidence, it was Boston Scientific's day.

Their technician happened to be downstairs in the operating room complex and was able to come up fairly quickly. She looked at the monitor.

Her first words were exactly the same.

"Oh shit."

That did not inspire confidence.

She stepped away to consult with someone. About thirty minutes later she returned.

"Are you able to stay here today and take nothing by mouth?"

"Yes," I said cautiously.

"We need to replace your ICD immediately."

That came as quite a shock. I had not realised the situation was heading toward full operating-room surgery. But when the device that may need to keep your heart beating needs attention, there is really only one sensible response.

So I agreed and waited.

And waited.

I had arrived around 9:30 in the morning. By mid-afternoon a nurse came to see me.

"Mr. Mittler, we're terribly sorry, but we can't do the surgery today. You'll have to come back tomorrow."

(Hmmm, another Arrhythmia Lab déjà vu?)

Under normal circumstances that would have been merely inconvenient.

But at the time I was deeply involved in preparations for MG 2022 — a major car convention in Peterborough that I was helping organise. More than two hundred cars were expected from across North America. The timing could not have been worse.

Then they added another complication.

After the procedure I would not be allowed to drive.

And if they had to replace the leads — the wires attached to the heart — my driver's licence could be suspended for six weeks.

We were only five weeks away from the convention.

Trying to manage an event of that size without being able to drive myself around was deeply unsettling. But there was no real choice. When the device that you might need to keep your heart beating ,needs attention, you listen.

So I went home and returned the next morning.

At nine o'clock sharp I was taken into a full operating theatre.

When the surgeon came in, I asked a simple question.

"Could you do this under local anaesthetic? Like a dentist — open the pocket, swap the device, sew it back up?"

She smiled. (well, she was masked but her voice smiled)

"Yes, we can do that."

"Good," I said. "Then I won't spend the day recovering from a general anaesthetic."

Then I asked the question that mattered most.

"What about the six weeks without driving?"

She explained that if the leads did not need to be touched — if they only replaced the ICD generator — she could notify the Ministry of Transportation and my licence would remain valid.

Halfway through the procedure she said,

"Mr. Mittler, your wires are fine. We only need to replace the device."

In other words, just the generator — the battery pack.

"You'll be good to go — and you won't have to stop driving."

That was an enormous relief.

It was yet another reminder that my cardiac and diabetic conditions continued to shape the boundaries of recovery — quietly present in the background of everyday life.

Five weeks later MG 2022 went ahead as planned. Almost two hundred cars arrived in Peterborough from across North America, and the convention was widely considered a success. It was my third time chairing or co-chairing a national MG convention — and, as it turned out, the last one I would ever lead.

I did not emerge from this experience with certainty or neatly resolved answers. What I gained instead was awareness — of timing, of people, of moments when intervention truly matters.

I became more attentive to the quiet signals: the subtle shifts that precede crisis, the early signs that something is changing. Those signals are easy to dismiss. I had dismissed them before.

What changed was not my understanding of mortality, but my relationship to it.

This story is not about escaping death. That was never the point.

It is about recognising the narrow windows where change is possible — medically, personally, humanly — and having the courage to act while those windows are still open.

Resetting the compass did not give me a destination.
It gave me direction.
And everything that followed depended on that.
Because the moment to act had not yet passed.
Because the window was still open.

Because it was not yet too late.

Epilogue – Life After

Survival does not return life to its previous settings. It changes the operating conditions.

Travel, once effortless, now requires planning of a different order. I carry more medical supplies than clothing: continuous glucose monitors, sensors, backup sensors, insulin, emergency glucose, medications for my heart, medications to compensate for organs I no longer have. Everything is counted. Everything is redundant. Nothing is optional.

Some vaccinations are no longer available to me. Yellow fever, for example, is off the table—too risky for someone without a spleen and with my medical history. That single limitation quietly redraws maps and alters itineraries in ways most travellers never need to consider.

Travel insurance is more expensive now. Pacemakers, cardiac history, complex medication regimens—all of it lives in fine print and underwriting tables. Coverage still exists, but it comes with questions, documentation, and cost.

Airports are their own choreography. I cannot pass through standard security scanners. I am patted down instead. Medical devices prompt explanations and letters from doctors. Supplies invite inspection. It is rarely hostile, but it is always visible. Privacy gives way to procedure. Apple juice is taboo on most flights, but I carry it with permission. Sharps? My wife had her sewing scissors confiscated while I take on hypodermic needles.

And yet, I still travel.

I walk new streets. I sit in unfamiliar cafés. I watch light change over water and mountains and cities far from home. I plan carefully, move deliberately, and rest when needed. The pace is different, but the curiosity remains intact.

What I lost was the illusion of invulnerability. What I gained was perspective.

Life after is not smaller. It is more intentional. It is shaped by limits, yes—but also by gratitude, attention, and a deeper awareness of what it means to be present.

I did not outrun time.
I learned to respect it.
And I am still here.
Thriving in Australia.

But that is another story.

A Message to the Reader

Does this sound familiar? The fatigue that doesn't lift, the discomfort that's easy to explain away, the quiet sense that something isn't right—I want you to hear this clearly:

- You are not imagining it.
- Do you eat antacids after any meal that has tomato sauce?
- Does a glass of wine upset your stomach?
- Does fatty food make you burp?
- Are you experiencing unusually strong-smelling flatulence and stools?
- How about a feeling of being full after only a small meal?
- Pain under your left rib cage?

I did not wake up one morning knowing my life was in danger. I rationalised symptoms. I adjusted routines. I waited. I told myself I would deal with things later—when they were clearer, when they were worse, when there was time.

What I learned is that clarity often arrives late. Windows close quietly. The body does not always announce urgency in ways that are easy to hear.

This book is not a warning meant to frighten you. It is an invitation to pay attention. To trust persistent signals. To ask harder questions. To push for answers when reassurance feels thin.

Intervention—medical, personal, human—works best when it happens early. Courage is not stoicism. Sometimes it is insisting on being taken seriously, even when it feels uncomfortable.

If this story prompts you to act sooner, speak up, seek another opinion, or simply listen more closely to your body, then it has done its work.

The Incredible Medical Team

I was fortunate to live in Ontario, where the estimated $1.1 million in medical expenses required to save my life were covered by the Ontario Health Insurance Plan. Just as important as the funding was the extraordinary team of doctors, specialists, and educators who, collectively, steered me through one of the most difficult periods of my life. I am forever grateful to each of them.

Mr. Grigori Dorfman, Surgeon – Perth, Australia
The doctor who, during a visit to Perth, first recognised the pancreatitis and warned me that it needed to be thoroughly investigated.

Dr. Larry Bacher, General Practitioner, Scarborough, Ontario
My long-term GP, who always had my best interests at heart and moved mountains to arrange timely testing and referrals.

Dr. Tim Devlin, Gastroenterologist, Scarborough, Ontario
A colleague of Larry's, who immediately referred me to a leading specialist.

Dr. Gary May, Gastroenterologist and Endoscopic Ultrasound Specialist – St. Michael's Hospital, Toronto.
The physician who tested, cleared me, tested again, and ultimately helped bring the situation into focus, making clear the seriousness of the choices ahead. I am especially grateful to Dr Gary May, whose clear guidance and timely advice helped me understand the urgency of my situation and act while there was still time.

Dr. Karanicolas, Surgeon – Sunnybrook Hospital, Toronto.
The doctor who carefully coached me, together with his fellow, on what to expect as a brittle diabetic and prepared me for what lay ahead before transferring the

surgery to his colleague.

Dr. Natalie Cockburn, Surgeon – Sunnybrook Hospital, Toronto.
Undertook a complex pancreatectomy that was expected to last four hours but extended to seven due to major complications—and brought it to a successful outcome.

Dr. Gideon Cohen, MD, MSc, PhD, FRCS(C) - Sunnybrook Hospital, Toronto.
Took over my case when the cardiac infarction occurred and guided the next critical phase of treatment.

Dr. Harindra Wijeysundera, MD, FRCPC - Sunnybrook Hospital, Toronto.
Head of Cardiac Care at Sunnybrook, who ultimately decided I was salvageable and that the team would work to make me a success story—and a survivor.

Dr. Angela Assal, Endocrinologist - Sunnybrook Hospital, Toronto.
Led the team that managed my diabetic care while I was in the Schulich Heart Institute.

SUNDEC – Sunnybrook Hospital Endocrinology Clinic, Toronto.
The team who monitored and managed my diabetes during recovery.

Jill Zweig and Leigh Caplan – Diabetes Educators, SUNDEC, Toronto.
Who patiently coached me on the use of insulin pens and later on transitioning to my Tandem t:slim insulin pump.

Dr. Andrew Yadegari, Cardiologist, Ajax, Ontario
Who monitored and coached me after my release from hospital and before our move to Australia.

Type 1 Family Diabetes Centre – Perth
Who took over my diabetic education and helped me to transition to a new GP, endocrinologist, and cardiologist in Australia. I learned a lot from these people and especially their podcast "Life in Beta". I hope it comes back.

Beck Newton – Type 1 Family Diabetes Centre, Perth
Who steered me through the myriad of landmines involved with Medicare, the NDSS, and the process of finding new doctors after we arrived in Perth. She also was a great mentor and counsel when I needed it. Thank you Beck.

Dr. Joey Kaye, Perth
Who continues to review me each year with quiet reassurance: "See you next year—keep doing whatever you're doing."

Dr. Peter Purnell, Joondalup
Who immediately placed me on a cardiac monitor after my arrival in Australia and who, with reassuring consistency, also says, "See you in a year."

Dexcom and Tandem
The technology companies whom I chose to manage my glucose monitoring and insulin dosing through. Not always perfect but if there was ever a time to be a diabetic (there is never a good time to be a diabetic) then this is it. I wake up in the morning nearly every morning at 6.1 mm/l. Who could ask for more?

I owe my life not to one person, but to a chain of skill, judgment, and care—each link essential, each decision made at the right time.

A Verse from Joyous Moments

Joyous Moments, when they call you with a date
Joyous Moments, let's make sure we're not too late
Joyous Moments, because, their work will save your life
Joyous Moments, salvation from the strife!

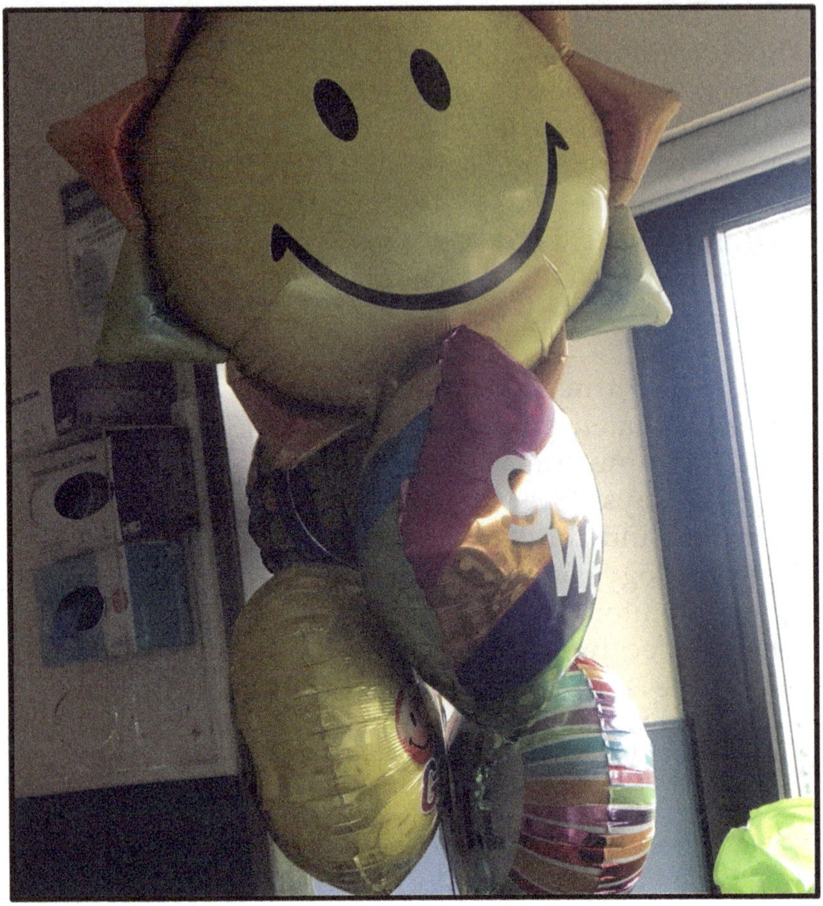

Photo 16: It's been a tough slog. But I prefer that to the alternative, so "Thank you, Lord, for thinking about me. I'm alive and doing fine."

[Signs 1970] That memorable line was composed by Les Emmerson, the lead singer and guitarist of the Canadian rock group Five Man Electrical Band.

Appendix A: Questions I Now Know to Ask

These appendices are included for readers who want practical takeaways from my experience. The questions below are ones I now know I should have asked much earlier.

"Why is the pancreatic duct dilated if there's no tumour?"
"What is pancreatitis?"

A dilated duct is not a diagnosis, but it is not normal either. I did not initially understand that the absence of a visible tumour does not mean the absence of disease. Asking this question earlier would have helped me understand how concerned my doctors already were.

In my case, the dilation was caused by an **IPMN (Intraductal Papillary Mucinous Neoplasm)** located at the neck of the pancreatic duct, near where it joins the bile duct. This growth produces mucous and can obstruct the duct, preventing digestive enzymes from flowing normally into the intestine.

The pancreas produces enzymes that help digest fats, proteins, and dairy. Normally, these enzymes are safely carried through the duct and activated in the intestine. When they cannot flow out properly, they can begin to damage the pancreas itself, leading to **acute pancreatitis**. Repeated attacks can lead to **chronic pancreatitis**.

I now understand why Mr. Dorfman was so careful to explain that in the spring of 2018 he was seeing **acute**, not chronic, pancreatitis.

"What does waiting cost me if cancer appears?"

Waiting is not neutral. Disease progresses even when symptoms are quiet. This question reframes "watch and

Types of diabetes explained

This book would be a disservice to us diabetics if I didn't try to distinguish between them. Many people have experienced unintended barbs and comments from uneducated non-diabetics. This is/was ME (*In italics*)

Feature	Type 1 Diabetes	Type 2 Diabetes	*Type 3c Diabetes (Pancreatogenic)*
Primary cause	Autoimmune destruction of insulin-producing beta cells	Insulin resistance with gradual beta-cell decline	Damage or removal of pancreas (pancreatectomy, *pancreatitis*, cancer, cysts, IPMN, trauma)
Insulin production	Little or none	Often present early, decreases over time	Little or *none*
Need for insulin	Always required	Sometimes required	Usually required or *insulin dependent*
Digestive enzyme production	Normal	Normal	Often reduced or *absent.*
Need for pancreatic enzymes	No	No	Often yes or *always (8 per day)*
Glucagon production	Reduced	Usually normal	Often reduced or *absent*
Risk of hypoglycemia (Low blood glucose)	Moderate–high	Lower unless using insulin	*Often high but very 'brittle' – high/low/high*
Blood sugar variability	Variable	Often more stable early	*Often highly variable. Brittle*
Body weight pattern	Often lean at diagnosis	Often overweight or insulin-resistant	Often weight loss or difficulty maintaining weight. *I am steady*
Onset	Usually younger age	Usually adulthood	*After pancreatic disease or surgery*
Digestive symptoms	Rare	Rare	Common *Indigestion, flatulence*
Management complexity	High	Variable	*Often very high*
Monitoring required	Frequent	Variable	*Frequent and intensive*

We have been on about 5 cruises since my pancreatic surgery. I cannot be x-rayed (pacemaker) wanded or scanned and I carry my 'pancreas' in a backpack wherever I go. I never leave home without it. I have a checklist I use before leaving with it. I have Doctors letters permitting sharps and juice to fly with me.

ITEM	WHY CARRY IT?
Insulin	Infusion set, syringe, pens (emergency to fill pump)
Juice	For Hypos 15 min recovery
Dex 4 Glucose Tabs	For Hypos 15 min recovery
Water	Hydration important
Squeeze Ball	Stress + strengthen L hand
Glucose Kit, meter, lances, plunger, spare batteries	Finger Sticks for Glucose checking. Backup for Dexcom CGM
Power Bank & cables	Charge phone and insulin pump if needed
Alcohol Swabs	For finger sticks & CGM changes
Dexcom Transmitter	Spare in case
Meds and List	AM & PM meds
Medical Tape Roll	Affixes pump tubing to skin
Hand Sanitizer	When sites and CGM change
T-slim tank cartridge	To replenish tank insulin
Insulin Pens	15 day supply carried
Insulin Pen Nibs	In case pump fails and need Manual dosing

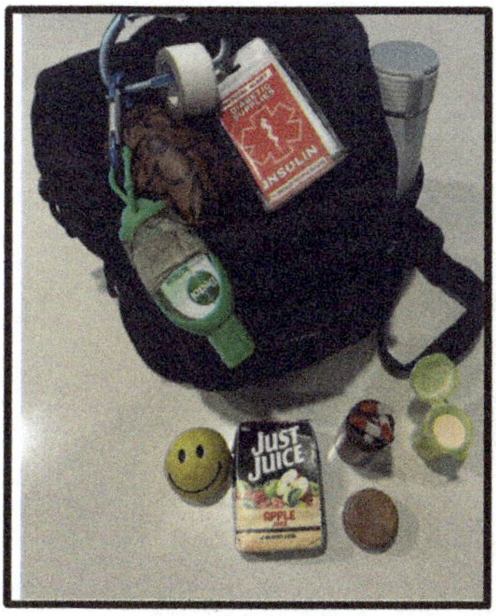

Photo 17: Pancreas pouch

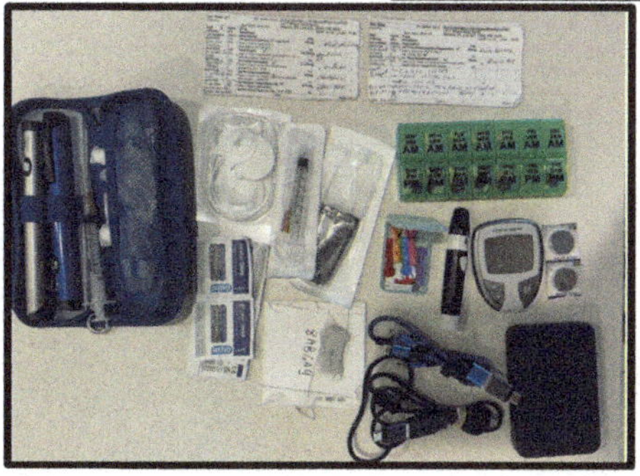

Photo 18: Everything I need to treat a Hypo or a Hyper

Appendix B: Warning Signs That Were Easy to Minimise

Looking back, several warning signs seemed small at the time but were not small in reality.

- **Recurrent pancreatitis without clear cause**
  Repeated inflammation is a signal, even when each episode resolves.

- **Unexpected weight loss**

- **Increasing duct dilation**
  Numbers changing slowly over time can be more important than a single result.

- **"Come back in six months" with worsening imaging**
  Time intervals can give a false sense of safety.

- **Being told "no cancer" without discussion of risk trajectory**
  Absence of cancer today is not the same as absence of risk tomorrow.

- **Gradually worsening digestive symptoms before my final visit with Dr. May (Spring 2020)**
  In the months leading up to that appointment, I began experiencing increasing acid indigestion and was taking antacids more frequently. I noticed more burping, stomach cramps, and bowel cramps. I also had increased flatulence, a bloated abdomen, and disrupted sleep.

Individually, each symptom seemed minor and easy to explain away. Together, they were a pattern I did not recognise soon enough.

Appendix C: So Now You're a "brittle diabetic"?

Living with 'brittle' diabetes

This appendix is written for readers who may one day face pancreatic surgery or insulin-dependent diabetes and want an honest picture of what daily life can look like afterward.

Important disclaimer:

Every person's insulin needs and responses are different. I am not going to suggest any dosing models here. I will simply explain how difficult my own carb-to-insulin ratio is to manage. You must seek the care and advice of an endocrinologist, a diabetes educator, or your GP and not rely on this book or online discussion groups for medical guidance.

"Brittle" is not a term used much in modern endocrinology, a fellow working with Dr. Karanicolas told me when preparing me for life after a pancreatectomy.

But then he added that this is exactly how my blood sugar would behave.

My target range is between **4 and 10 mmol/L** (millimoles of glucose per litre of blood).

For American readers, multiply those numbers by 18 to get **72 to 180 mg/dL**.

So what does that mean in daily life?

Normally, the body—with its pancreas, insulin, and enzymes—begins handling digestion automatically.

But not in Type 1 or Type 3c diabetes.

Blood sugar can change quickly and unpredictably. It requires attention, planning, and constant adjustment. It is manageable—but it demands respect.

Insulin becomes your life-dependent friend and enemy at the same time: something you rely on, something you must handle carefully, something you must never forget. You keep it cool but never frozen. You pack it carefully in your luggage. On long flights, you sometimes ask a flight attendant to store it safely—and you never forget to retrieve it before landing.

It is pressure.

It is exhausting.

But it is life.

Monitoring and dosing

My finger-stick glucose meter and my Dexcom continuous glucose monitor tell me where my blood sugar is at that moment and which direction it is moving.

By knowing how much insulin is already in my body (IOB), my carb-to-insulin ratio, and the amount of carbohydrate I am about to eat, I can calculate how much insulin to bolus.

Sugars act quickly. They are what I use to recover from hypoglycaemia.

But carbohydrates—those are the real challenge.

Counting carbs is time-consuming and frustrating, and the results are never perfectly predictable. The same food can affect me differently from one day to the next depending on activity, stress, illness, or timing.

Today a slice of bread might raise my glucose by 4 mmol/L. Tomorrow, after a walk or some gardening, the effect may be very different.

Time in Range and Unpredictability

Some sources list more than forty factors that can affect blood glucose levels - forty-two factors, in fact.

That means there are **42 factorial** possible combinations influencing what my dose should be—decisions that must often be made fifteen minutes before I eat.

42! equals:

1,405,006,117,752,879,898,543,142,606,244,511,569,936,384,000,000,000

A number so large it hardly means anything in practical terms—except this:

Getting it exactly right every time is impossible.

Sometimes it feels like a crap shoot.

But it is the reality many people with Type 1 or Type 3c diabetes live with every day.

Enzymes and Digestion

Eating is no longer automatic. Enzymes become part of every meal, and timing matters. Over time, this becomes routine—but it is a real adjustment.

Earlier I told the story of disagreeing with a nurse who insisted I take CREON after I had eaten. I will not repeat that here, but I will say this:

I keep a substantial reserve of CREON because I am genuinely afraid of shortages. These enzymes are derived from porcine pancreas, so supply ultimately depends on agricultural production.

Without CREON, food does not digest properly. I bloat, cramp, and produce enough gas to clear Yankee Stadium in one blast. Humour aside, this is simply part of life for people living without a pancreas.

What recovery really looks like

Recovery was not dramatic or heroic. It was slow, uneven, and measured in small gains—walking a little farther, eating a little more, sleeping a little better. Progress often looked ordinary, but it was meaningful.

One unexpected truth is this: I no longer live with the fear of pancreatic cancer. That particular risk is gone. That brings a certain peace.

Something else may come someday. That is life. But I do not spend my time worrying about a future I almost did not have.

Think about that for a moment.

I am lucky, blessed, and grateful to be here.

And if something else comes along, I will deal with it too—

Hopefully before it is not too late.

Appendix D: Songs from the Journey

During my time in hospital, music became both an outlet and a way to process what was happening around me. The following songs were written during that period.

Desperate Man

Written during COVID-19 while watching news reports of people losing jobs, businesses, and security. The song reflects the broader anxiety and hardship of that time. It began as a song of self-pity, but I soon realised that many people were far worse off than I was. While recovering in the Schulich Heart Institute, I reshaped it into the version that appears on Spotify.

Hurry Up and Wait: Bumped Again

This song was inspired by the repeated delays in my discharge while waiting for an ICD, after being bumped from the list for ten consecutive days. The song captures the frustration and dark humour of that experience.

Joyous Moments

A reflection on gratitude and the unexpected blessings that can arrive when life intervenes before it is too late.

Angels in Blue

A tribute to the nurses whose skill, compassion, and professionalism brought both care and comfort during my hospitalisation.

Echoes of Angels in Blue

A remix of Angels in Blue, created using an AI music generator (Songer). I wanted to explore whether my lyrics and a model of my voice could be placed into a newly generated musical setting. The results pleasantly surprised me and encouraged me to continue experimenting and creating.

Music during this time was more than a pastime—it helped me stay grounded, process fear, and remind myself that I was still alive and still creating.

Use the QR code link to the songs referred to in this book

Photo 18: Scan to see the lyrics and hear the music

https://hyperfollow.com/beforeitwastoolate

Thank you for reading the book and listening to my music.